LOW FODMAP COOKBOOK

30 Days of Delicious Low FODMAP Meals Made Easy

T. John

COPYRIGHT PAGE

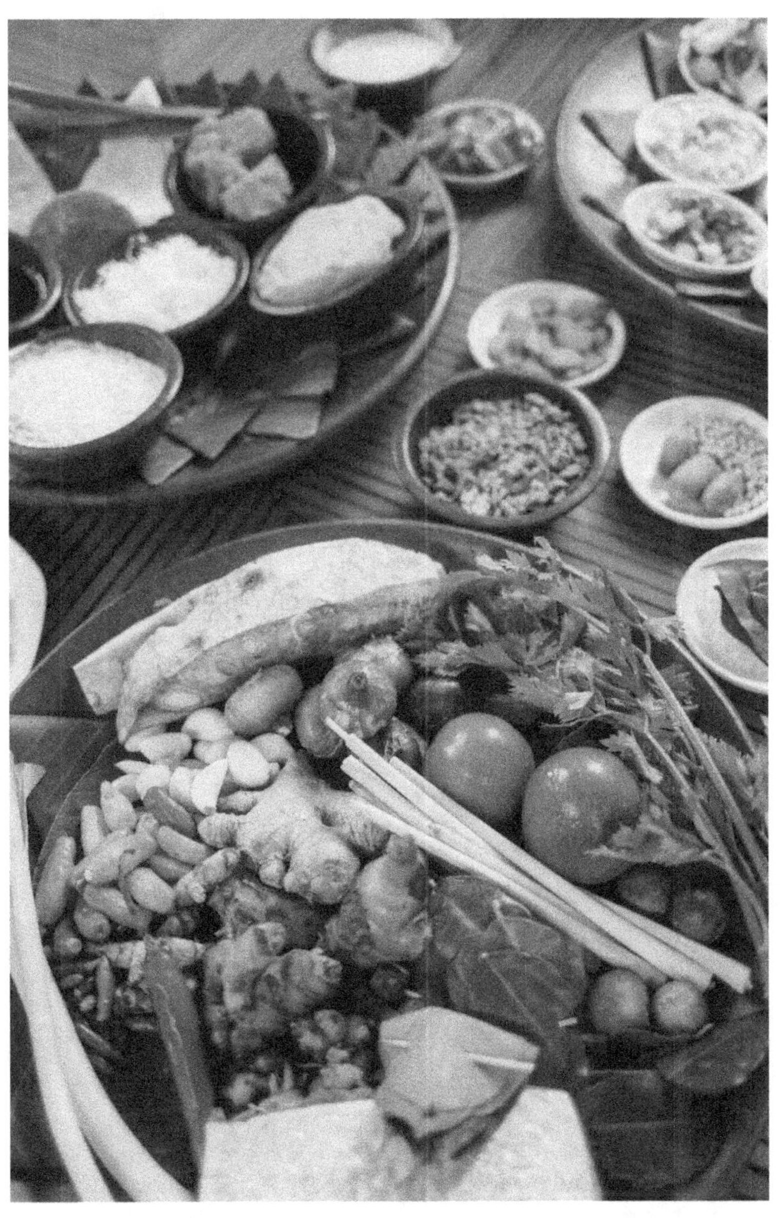

TABLE OF CONTENTS

Chapter 5: Snacks and Appetizers 80

INTRODUCTION

Forget the latest fad diets or the allure of quick fixes. The low FODMAP diet isn't a trendy flash in the pan; it's a targeted approach to managing gut issues like irritable bowel syndrome (IBS). But navigating the world of FODMAPs (Fermentable Oligosaccharides, Disaccharides, Monols and Polyols) can feel like deciphering an ancient language. Fear not, fellow gut warriors! This guide will be your Rosetta Stone, helping you understand the "what," "why," and "how" of the low FODMAP diet, all with a healthy dose of real-life insights.

The Lowdown on FODMAPs: Imagine tiny sugar molecules in certain foods that your gut isn't too keen on digesting. These FODMAPs attract water, leading to bloating, gas, and other unpleasantries. The low FODMAP diet aims to minimize these troublemakers, giving your gut a much-needed break.

Benefits Beyond Belief: While managing IBS is the main focus, the low FODMAP diet can offer surprising perks. Many people report reduced anxiety, improved sleep, and even clearer skin! It's like a gut reset that ripples outwards, bringing a newfound sense of wellbeing.

The Food Flip Side: Now, the fun (and sometimes frustrating) part: figuring out what to eat and what to avoid. Think of it as an adventure, not a restriction! Embrace the bounty of low FODMAP delights like leafy greens, lean protein, and naturally sweet fruits like berries. Befriend herbs and spices for added flavor, and don't forget the power of a good homemade soup.

But Wait, There's More: The low FODMAP diet isn't a one-size-fits-all solution. What works for one person might not be the magic bullet for another. Listen to your body, experiment with different foods, and keep a food diary to track your gut's reactions. Remember, it's a journey, not a destination.

Considerations for the Cautious: Before embarking on this gut-friendly quest, consult a healthcare professional or registered dietitian. They can tailor the diet to your specific needs and provide guidance on reintroducing FODMAPs later on.

The Final FODMAP Word: The low FODMAP diet isn't just about food; it's about reclaiming control of your gut and your wellbeing. It's a commitment, but the rewards can be life-changing. So, grab your curiosity, a healthy dose of patience, and dive into the world of FODMAPs. Your gut will thank you for it!

Bonus Tip: Don't go it alone! Join online communities or support groups to connect with others on the low FODMAP journey. Sharing tips, recipes, and encouragement can make all the difference.

Remember, understanding the low FODMAP diet is key to unlocking its potential benefits. Approach it with an open mind, a dash of experimentation, and a whole lot of self-compassion. Your gut will be your guide, leading you towards a happier, healthier you, one delicious bite at a time.

Chapter 1: 30 Day Meal Plan

Week 1:

Day 1:

- Breakfast: Quinoa Breakfast Bowl
- Lunch: Chicken and Vegetable Stir-Fry
- Dinner: Lemon Herb Baked Cod
- Snack: Parmesan Zucchini Chips
- Dessert: Chocolate Avocado Mousse

Day 2:

- Breakfast: Spinach and Feta Omelette
- Lunch: Grilled Shrimp Salad with Citrus Dressing
- Dinner: Beef and Vegetable Stir-Fry
- Snack: Deviled Eggs with Chives
- Dessert: Almond Flour Banana Bread

Day 3:

- Breakfast: Blueberry Almond Smoothie Bowl
- Lunch: Quinoa and Roasted Vegetable Bowl

- Dinner: Cilantro Lime Chicken with Quinoa

- Snack: Greek Yogurt and Dill Dip

- Dessert: Berry and Coconut Ice Pops

Day 4:

- Breakfast: Banana Pancakes (with Gluten-Free Flour)

- Lunch: Turkey and Cranberry Wrap (Gluten-Free)

- Dinner: Eggplant Parmesan (Gluten-Free)

- Snack: Buffalo Chicken Wings

- Dessert: Lemon Sorbet

Day 5:

- Breakfast: Chia Seed Pudding with Berries

- Lunch: Caprese Salad with Balsamic Glaze

- Dinner: Shrimp and Asparagus Risotto

- Snack: Mozzarella and Tomato Skewers

- Dessert: Pumpkin Pie Bites

Day 6:

- Breakfast: Avocado and Tomato Breakfast Wrap

- Lunch: Lentil and Vegetable Soup
- Dinner: Grilled Pork Chops with Rosemary Potatoes
- Snack: Roasted Chickpeas
- Dessert: Chocolate-Dipped Strawberries

Day 7:

- Breakfast: Zucchini and Bacon Egg Muffins
- Lunch: Tuna Salad Lettuce Wraps
- Dinner: Zucchini Noodles with Pesto
- Snack: Hummus with Carrot Sticks
- Dessert: Vanilla Chia Seed Pudding

Week 2:

Day 8:

- Breakfast: Smoked Salmon and Cream Cheese Bagel (Gluten-Free)
- Lunch: Roasted Red Pepper and Feta Quiche (Gluten-Free Crust)
- Dinner: Moroccan Spiced Chicken Skewers
- Snack: Cheese and Grape Plate
- Dessert: Coconut Macaroons

Day 9:

- Breakfast: Orange Ginger Infused Quinoa Porridge
- Lunch: Pesto Chicken and Tomato Skewers
- Dinner: Teriyaki Salmon with Brown Rice
- Snack: Bacon-Wrapped Jalapeño Poppers
- Dessert: Kiwi and Pineapple Fruit Salad

Day 10:

- Breakfast: Greek Yogurt Parfait with Low FODMAP Fruits
- Lunch: Spaghetti Squash with Pesto and Cherry Tomatoes
- Dinner: Chicken and Broccoli Casserole (Gluten-Free)
- Snack: Guacamole with Bell Pepper Strips
- Dessert: Raspberry Almond Cake (Gluten-Free)

Day 11:

- Breakfast: Turkey Sausage and Potato Hash
- Lunch: Greek Salad with Grilled Chicken
- Dinner: Spinach and Ricotta Stuffed Chicken Breast
- Snack: Cucumber and Feta Bites

- Dessert: Mint Chocolate Chip Cookies

Day 12:

- Breakfast: Peanut Butter and Banana Toast (Gluten-Free Bread)
- Lunch: Eggplant and Mozzarella Stack
- Dinner: Vegetable and Tofu Curry
- Snack: Mixed Nuts and Seeds
- Dessert: Orange Sorbet

Day 13:

- Breakfast: Raspberry Coconut Breakfast Bars
- Lunch: Thai Chicken Lettuce Cups
- Dinner: Lemon Garlic Shrimp Scampi
- Snack: Olive Tapenade on Gluten-Free Crackers
- Dessert: Blueberry Yogurt Popsicles

Day 14:

- Breakfast: Breakfast Burrito with Scrambled Eggs and Salsa
- Lunch: Turkey and Avocado Sushi Rolls

- Dinner: Stuffed Bell Peppers with Ground Turkey
- Snack: Edamame with Sea Salt
- Dessert: Almond Butter Cups

Week 3:

Day 15:

- Breakfast: FODMAP-Friendly Apple Crisp
- Lunch: Pumpkin and Sage Risotto
- Dinner: BBQ Pulled Chicken Lettuce Wraps
- Snack: Smoked Salmon Pinwheels
- Dessert: Chocolate Avocado Mousse

Day 16:

- Breakfast: Almond Flour Banana Bread
- Lunch: Chicken and Vegetable Stir-Fry
- Dinner: Lemon Herb Baked Cod
- Snack: Parmesan Zucchini Chips
- Dessert: Berry and Coconut Ice Pops

Day 17:

- Breakfast: Blueberry Almond Smoothie Bowl

- Lunch: Grilled Shrimp Salad with Citrus Dressing
- Dinner: Beef and Vegetable Stir-Fry
- Snack: Deviled Eggs with Chives
- Dessert: Almond Butter Cups

Day 18:

- Breakfast: Banana Pancakes (with Gluten-Free Flour)
- Lunch: Turkey and Cranberry Wrap (Gluten-Free)
- Dinner: Eggplant Parmesan (Gluten-Free)
- Snack: Buffalo Chicken Wings
- Dessert: Lemon Sorbet

Day 19:

- Breakfast: Chia Seed Pudding with Berries
- Lunch: Caprese Salad with Balsamic Glaze
- Dinner: Shrimp and Asparagus Risotto
- Snack: Mozzarella and Tomato Skewers
- Dessert: Pumpkin Pie Bites

Day 20:

- Breakfast: Avocado and Tomato Breakfast Wrap
- Lunch: Lentil and Vegetable Soup
- Dinner: Grilled Pork Chops with Rosemary Potatoes
- Snack: Roasted Chickpeas
- Dessert: Chocolate-Dipped Strawberries

Day 21:

- Breakfast: Zucchini and Bacon Egg Muffins
- Lunch: Tuna Salad Lettuce Wraps
- Dinner: Zucchini Noodles with Pesto
- Snack: Hummus with Carrot Sticks
- Dessert: Vanilla Chia Seed Pudding

Week 4

Day 22:

- Breakfast: Smoked Salmon and Cream Cheese Bagel (Gluten-Free)
- Lunch: Roasted Red Pepper and Feta Quiche (Gluten-Free Crust)
- Dinner: Moroccan Spiced Chicken Skewers

- Snack: Cheese and Grape Plate

- Dessert: Coconut Macaroons

Day 23:

- Breakfast: Orange Ginger Infused Quinoa Porridge

- Lunch: Pesto Chicken and Tomato Skewers

- Dinner: Teriyaki Salmon with Brown Rice

- Snack: Bacon-Wrapped Jalapeño Poppers

- Dessert: Kiwi and Pineapple Fruit Salad

Day 24:

- Breakfast: Greek Yogurt Parfait with Low FODMAP Fruits

- Lunch: Spaghetti Squash with Pesto and Cherry Tomatoes

- Dinner: Chicken and Broccoli Casserole (Gluten-Free)

- Snack: Guacamole with Bell Pepper Strips

- Dessert: Raspberry Almond Cake (Gluten-Free)

Day 25:

- Breakfast: Turkey Sausage and Potato Hash
- Lunch: Greek Salad with Grilled Chicken
- Dinner: Spinach and Ricotta Stuffed Chicken Breast
- Snack: Cucumber and Feta Bites
- Dessert: Mint Chocolate Chip Cookies

Day 26:

- Breakfast: Peanut Butter and Banana Toast (Gluten-Free Bread)
- Lunch: Eggplant and Mozzarella Stack
- Dinner: Vegetable and Tofu Curry
- Snack: Mixed Nuts and Seeds
- Dessert: Orange Sorbet

Day 27:

- Breakfast: Raspberry Coconut Breakfast Bars
- Lunch: Thai Chicken Lettuce Cups
- Dinner: Lemon Garlic Shrimp Scampi
- Snack: Olive Tapenade on Gluten-Free Crackers
- Dessert: Blueberry Yogurt Popsicles

Day 28:

- Breakfast: Breakfast Burrito with Scrambled Eggs and Salsa
- Lunch: Turkey and Avocado Sushi Rolls
- Dinner: Stuffed Bell Peppers with Ground Turkey
- Snack: Edamame with Sea Salt
- Dessert: Almond Butter Cups

Day 29:

- Breakfast: FODMAP-Friendly Apple Crisp
- Lunch: Pumpkin and Sage Risotto
- Dinner: BBQ Pulled Chicken Lettuce Wraps
- Snack: Smoked Salmon Pinwheels
- Dessert: Chocolate Avocado Mousse

Day 30:

- Breakfast: Almond Flour Banana Bread
- Lunch: Chicken and Vegetable Stir-Fry
- Dinner: Lemon Herb Baked Cod
- Snack: Parmesan Zucchini Chips
- Dessert: Berry and Coconut Ice Pops

Chapter 2: Breakfast Recipes

This chapter is a treasure trove of morning goodness, offering you a variety of flavorful options to kickstart your day. From wholesome grains to protein-packed treats, each recipe is crafted to align with your dietary needs.

Quinoa Breakfast Bowl

Ingredients:

- 1 cup cooked quinoa
- 1/4 cup sliced strawberries
- 1 tablespoon chopped almonds
- 1 tablespoon maple syrup
- 1/2 teaspoon vanilla extract

Instructions:

1. In a bowl, combine quinoa, strawberries, and almonds.
2. Drizzle with maple syrup and vanilla extract.
3. Gently toss and enjoy!

Nutrition Information:

- Calories: 300
- Protein: 8g
- Carbohydrates: 45g
- Fat: 10g
- Fiber: 6g
- Sugar: 8g
- Portion Size: 1 bowl

Spinach and Feta Omelette

Ingredients:

- 2 large eggs
- 1/4 cup spinach, chopped
- 2 tablespoons crumbled feta cheese
- Salt and pepper to taste

Instructions:

1. Whisk eggs and pour into a heated, greased pan.
2. Add spinach and feta on one half of the omelette.
3. Fold the other half over the fillings, cook until set, and serve.

Nutrition Information:

- Calories: 220
- Protein: 14g
- Carbohydrates: 2g
- Fat: 18g
- Fiber: 1g
- Sugar: 0g
- Portion Size: 1 omelette

Blueberry Almond Smoothie Bowl

Ingredients:

- 1 cup blueberries (fresh or frozen)
- 1/2 banana
- 1/4 cup almond butter
- 1 cup almond milk
- Ice cubes (optional)

Instructions:

1. Blend blueberries, banana, almond butter, and almond milk until smooth.

2. Pour into a bowl and top with your favorite low FODMAP toppings.

Nutrition Information:

- Calories: 320
- Protein: 8g
- Carbohydrates: 30g
- Fat: 20g
- Fiber: 7g
- Sugar: 15g
- Portion Size: 1 bowl

Banana Pancakes (with Gluten-Free Flour)

Ingredients:

- 1 ripe banana, mashed
- 1/2 cup gluten-free flour
- 1/2 teaspoon baking powder
- 1/4 cup lactose-free milk
- 1 tablespoon maple syrup

Instructions:

1. Mix banana, gluten-free flour, baking powder, and milk.
2. Cook spoonfuls of batter on a hot griddle until golden.
3. Drizzle with maple syrup and serve.

Nutrition Information:

- Calories: 260
- Protein: 5g
- Carbohydrates: 45g
- Fat: 7g
- Fiber: 3g
- Sugar: 12g
- Portion Size: 2 pancakes

Chia Seed Pudding with Berries

Ingredients:

- 2 tablespoons chia seeds
- 1/2 cup lactose-free milk
- 1/4 teaspoon vanilla extract

- Mixed berries for topping

Instructions:

1. Mix chia seeds, milk, and vanilla extract. Refrigerate overnight.
2. Top with mixed berries before serving.

Nutrition Information:

- Calories: 180
- Protein: 5g
- Carbohydrates: 20g
- Fat: 9g
- Fiber: 8g
- Sugar: 5g
- Portion Size: 1 serving

Avocado and Tomato Breakfast Wrap

Ingredients:

- 1 gluten-free wrap
- 1/2 avocado, sliced

- 1/2 cup cherry tomatoes, halved
- Salt and pepper to taste

Instructions:

1. Lay out the gluten-free wrap.
2. Arrange avocado slices and cherry tomatoes.
3. Season with salt and pepper, wrap, and enjoy!

Nutrition Information:

- Calories: 280
- Protein: 5g
- Carbohydrates: 30g
- Fat: 15g
- Fiber: 8g
- Sugar: 3g
- Portion Size: 1 wrap

Zucchini and Bacon Egg Muffins

Ingredients:

- 4 large eggs
- 1/2 cup zucchini, grated

- 3 slices cooked bacon, crumbled
- 1/4 cup lactose-free milk

Instructions:

1. Preheat oven to 350°F (175°C).
2. Whisk eggs and mix with zucchini, bacon, and milk.
3. Pour into muffin cups and bake for 20 minutes.

Nutrition Information:

- Calories: 220
- Protein: 12g
- Carbohydrates: 3g
- Fat: 18g
- Fiber: 1g
- Sugar: 1g
- Portion Size: 2 muffins

Maple Cinnamon Oatmeal

Ingredients:

- 1/2 cup old-fashioned oats
- 1 cup lactose-free milk

- 1 tablespoon maple syrup
- 1/2 teaspoon ground cinnamon

Instructions:

1. Cook oats with milk according to package instructions.
2. Stir in maple syrup and cinnamon.
3. Serve warm.

Nutrition Information:

- Calories: 250
- Protein: 8g
- Carbohydrates: 40g
- Fat: 6g
- Fiber: 5g
- Sugar: 10g
- Portion Size: 1 serving

Smoked Salmon and Cream Cheese Bagel (Gluten-Free)

Ingredients:

- 1 gluten-free bagel
- 2 tablespoons lactose-free cream cheese
- 2 slices smoked salmon
- Capers and dill for garnish

Instructions:

1. Toast the gluten-free bagel.
2. Spread cream cheese on each half.
3. Top with smoked salmon, capers, and dill.

Nutrition Information:

- Calories: 320
- Protein: 18g
- Carbohydrates: 30g
- Fat: 15g
- Fiber: 3g
- Sugar: 2g
- Portion Size: 1 bagel

Orange Ginger Infused Quinoa Porridge

Ingredients:

- 1/2 cup cooked quinoa
- 1/2 cup lactose-free milk
- 1 tablespoon orange zest
- 1/2 teaspoon ground ginger
- 1 tablespoon maple syrup

Instructions:

1. Mix quinoa, milk, orange zest, and ginger.
2. Heat until warm, stirring occasionally.
3. Drizzle with maple syrup and serve.

Nutrition Information:

- Calories: 280
- Protein: 7g
- Carbohydrates: 45g
- Fat: 8g
- Fiber: 5g
- Sugar: 10g

- Portion Size: 1 serving

Greek Yogurt Parfait with Low FODMAP Fruits

Ingredients:

- 1 cup lactose-free Greek yogurt
- 1/2 cup strawberries, sliced
- 1/4 cup blueberries
- 2 tablespoons low FODMAP granola

Instructions:

1. In a glass, layer Greek yogurt, strawberries, blueberries, and granola.
2. Repeat the layers.
3. Finish with a sprinkle of granola on top.

Nutrition Information:

- Calories: 280
- Protein: 15g
- Carbohydrates: 35g
- Fat: 10g

- Fiber: 5g

- Sugar: 15g

- Portion Size: 1 parfait

Turkey Sausage and Potato Hash

Ingredients:

- 1/2 lb low FODMAP turkey sausage

- 2 cups potatoes, diced

- 1/2 cup bell peppers, chopped

- 1/4 cup green onions, sliced

- Salt and pepper to taste

Instructions:

1. Cook turkey sausage in a skillet until browned.

2. Add potatoes, bell peppers, and green onions.

3. Cook until potatoes are golden and serve.

Nutrition Information:

- Calories: 320

- Protein: 15g

- Carbohydrates: 30g

- Fat: 15g

- Fiber: 5g

- Sugar: 3g

- Portion Size: 1 serving

Peanut Butter and Banana Toast (Gluten-Free Bread)

Ingredients:

- 2 slices gluten-free bread

- 2 tablespoons peanut butter

- 1 banana, sliced

- Drizzle of honey (optional)

Instructions:

1. Toast gluten-free bread slices.

2. Spread peanut butter on each slice.

3. Top with banana slices and drizzle with honey.

Nutrition Information:

- Calories: 300

- Protein: 8g

- Carbohydrates: 45g

- Fat: 12g

- Fiber: 6g

- Sugar: 15g

- Portion Size: 1 serving

Raspberry Coconut Breakfast Bars

Ingredients:

- 1 cup gluten-free oats

- 1/2 cup almond flour

- 1/4 cup shredded coconut

- 1/2 cup raspberry jam (low FODMAP)

- 1/4 cup coconut oil, melted

Instructions:

1. Mix oats, almond flour, shredded coconut, and melted coconut oil.

2. Press half of the mixture into a baking dish.

3. Spread raspberry jam over the mixture.

4. Sprinkle the remaining oat mixture on top.

5. Bake until golden and let cool before cutting into bars.

Nutrition Information:

- Calories: 220
- Protein: 4g
- Carbohydrates: 30g
- Fat: 10g
- Fiber: 4g
- Sugar: 12g
- Portion Size: 1 bar

Breakfast Burrito with Scrambled Eggs and Salsa

Ingredients:

- 2 gluten-free tortillas
- 4 large eggs, scrambled
- 1/2 cup lactose-free cheddar cheese, shredded
- 1/4 cup salsa (low FODMAP)

Instructions:

1. Fill each tortilla with scrambled eggs, cheese, and salsa.

2. Roll into a burrito and serve.

Nutrition Information:

- Calories: 320
- Protein: 16g
- Carbohydrates: 25g
- Fat: 18g
- Fiber: 3g
- Sugar: 2g
- Portion Size: 1 burrito

Chapter 3: Lunch Recipes

Welcome to Chapter 3 of our Low FODMAP Cookbook, where we dive into a delightful array of Lunch Recipes designed to tantalize your taste buds while adhering to your dietary needs.

Chicken and Vegetable Stir-Fry

Ingredients:

- 1 lb chicken breast, sliced
- 2 cups broccoli florets
- 1 red bell pepper, sliced
- 1 zucchini, sliced
- 2 carrots, julienned
- 2 tablespoons low FODMAP stir-fry sauce

Instructions:

1. In a wok, stir-fry chicken until cooked.
2. Add vegetables and stir-fry until crisp-tender.

3. Pour in stir-fry sauce, toss, and cook for an additional 2 minutes.

4. Serve hot.

Nutrition Information (per serving):

- Calories: 300

- Protein: 25g

- Carbohydrates: 20g

- Fat: 12g

- Fiber: 5g

- Sugar: 6g

- Portion Size: 1.5 cups

Grilled Shrimp Salad with Citrus Dressing

Ingredients:

- 1 lb shrimp, peeled and deveined

- 6 cups mixed salad greens

- 1 cup cherry tomatoes, halved

- 1 avocado, diced

- 1/4 cup feta cheese, crumbled

- Citrus dressing

Instructions:

1. Grill shrimp until pink and opaque.

2. Toss salad greens, tomatoes, avocado, and shrimp.

3. Drizzle with citrus dressing, sprinkle with feta, and toss gently.

4. Serve chilled.

Nutrition Information (per serving):

- Calories: 280

- Protein: 20g

- Carbohydrates: 15g

- Fat: 18g

- Fiber: 8g

- Sugar: 4g

- Portion Size: 2 cups

Quinoa and Roasted Vegetable Bowl

Ingredients:

- 1 cup quinoa, cooked

- 2 cups mixed roasted vegetables (zucchini, bell peppers, eggplant)
- 1/4 cup fresh basil, chopped
- 2 tablespoons olive oil
- Salt and pepper to taste

Instructions:

1. Combine quinoa, roasted vegetables, and basil.
2. Drizzle with olive oil, season with salt and pepper.
3. Toss gently until well mixed.
4. Serve warm or at room temperature.

Nutrition Information (per serving):

- Calories: 320
- Protein: 10g
- Carbohydrates: 45g
- Fat: 12g
- Fiber: 8g
- Sugar: 3g
- Portion Size: 1.5 cups

Turkey and Cranberry Wrap (Gluten-Free)

Ingredients:

- 4 gluten-free tortillas
- 1 lb turkey breast, thinly sliced
- 1/2 cup cranberry sauce (low FODMAP)
- 2 cups mixed greens
- 1/4 cup walnuts, chopped

Instructions:

1. Lay out tortillas and layer with turkey, cranberry sauce, greens, and walnuts.
2. Roll tightly, slice in half, and secure with toothpicks.
3. Serve chilled or at room temperature.

Nutrition Information (per serving):

- Calories: 280
- Protein: 18g
- Carbohydrates: 30g
- Fat: 12g
- Fiber: 6g

- Sugar: 8g
- Portion Size: 1 wrap

Caprese Salad with Balsamic Glaze

Ingredients:

- 4 large tomatoes, sliced
- 1 lb fresh mozzarella, sliced
- Fresh basil leaves
- Balsamic glaze
- Salt and pepper to taste

Instructions:

1. Arrange tomato and mozzarella slices on a platter.
2. Tuck basil leaves between slices.
3. Drizzle with balsamic glaze, season with salt and pepper.
4. Serve immediately.

Nutrition Information (per serving):

- Calories: 250
- Protein: 15g

- Carbohydrates: 10g

- Fat: 18g

- Fiber: 3g

- Sugar: 5g

- Portion Size: 1 cup

Lentil and Vegetable Soup

Ingredients:

- 1 cup green lentils, rinsed

- 4 cups low FODMAP vegetable broth

- 2 carrots, diced

- 2 celery stalks, chopped

- 1 cup spinach, chopped

- 1 teaspoon cumin

- Salt and pepper to taste

Instructions:

1. In a pot, combine lentils, broth, carrots, and celery.

2. Simmer until lentils are tender.

3. Add spinach, cumin, salt, and pepper.

4. Cook for an additional 5 minutes.

5. Serve hot.

Nutrition Information (per serving):

- Calories: 220
- Protein: 14g
- Carbohydrates: 35g
- Fat: 2g
- Fiber: 12g
- Sugar: 3g
- Portion Size: 1.5 cups

Tuna Salad Lettuce Wraps

Ingredients:

- 2 cans tuna, drained
- 1/4 cup mayonnaise (low FODMAP)
- 1 celery stalk, finely chopped
- 1 tablespoon Dijon mustard
- Lettuce leaves for wrapping

Instructions:

1. In a bowl, mix tuna, mayonnaise, celery, and Dijon.

2. Spoon mixture onto lettuce leaves.

3. Roll and secure with toothpicks.

4. Serve chilled.

Nutrition Information (per serving):

- Calories: 180

- Protein: 20g

- Carbohydrates: 2g

- Fat: 10g

- Fiber: 1g

- Sugar: 0g

- Portion Size: 2 wraps

Roasted Red Pepper and Feta Quiche (Gluten-Free Crust)

Ingredients:

- 1 gluten-free pie crust

- 1 cup roasted red peppers, chopped

- 1 cup feta cheese, crumbled

- 6 large eggs

- 1 cup lactose-free milk

- Salt and pepper to taste

Instructions:

1. Preheat oven to 350°F (175°C).
2. Layer red peppers and feta in pie crust.
3. Whisk eggs, milk, salt, and pepper. Pour over the filling.
4. Bake for 30-35 minutes or until set.
5. Let it cool before slicing.

Nutrition Information (per serving):

- Calories: 280
- Protein: 14g
- Carbohydrates: 15g
- Fat: 18g
- Fiber: 2g
- Sugar: 3g
- Portion Size: 1 slice

Pesto Chicken and Tomato Skewers

Ingredients:

- 1 lb chicken breast, cut into chunks
- 1 cup cherry tomatoes
- 1/4 cup low FODMAP pesto
- Wooden skewers, soaked in water

Instructions:

1. Thread chicken and tomatoes onto skewers.
2. Brush with pesto and grill until chicken is cooked.
3. Serve hot.

Nutrition Information (per serving):

- Calories: 230
- Protein: 25g
- Carbohydrates: 5g
- Fat: 12g
- Fiber: 1g
- Sugar: 2g
- Portion Size: 2 skewers

Spaghetti Squash with Pesto and Cherry Tomatoes

Ingredients:

- 1 medium spaghetti squash
- 1/2 cup low FODMAP pesto
- 1 cup cherry tomatoes, halved
- Fresh basil for garnish

Instructions:

1. Roast spaghetti squash until tender.
2. Scrape the flesh into strands.
3. Toss with pesto and cherry tomatoes.
4. Garnish with fresh basil.
5. Serve warm.

Nutrition Information (per serving):

- Calories: 180
- Protein: 3g
- Carbohydrates: 20g
- Fat: 10g
- Fiber: 4g

- Sugar: 6g
- Portion Size: 1 cup

Greek Salad with Grilled Chicken

Ingredients:

- 1 lb chicken thighs, grilled and sliced
- 4 cups mixed salad greens
- 1 cup cucumber, sliced
- 1 cup cherry tomatoes, halved
- 1/2 cup Kalamata olives
- 1/4 cup feta cheese, crumbled
- Greek dressing

Instructions:

1. Toss salad greens, cucumber, tomatoes, olives, and grilled chicken.
2. Drizzle with Greek dressing and sprinkle with feta.
3. Serve chilled.

Nutrition Information (per serving):

- Calories: 320

- Protein: 22g

- Carbohydrates: 15g

- Fat: 18g

- Fiber: 6g

- Sugar: 5g

- Portion Size: 2 cups

Eggplant and Mozzarella Stack

Ingredients:

- 2 medium eggplants, sliced

- 1 cup mozzarella cheese, sliced

- 2 cups tomato sauce (low FODMAP)

- Fresh basil for garnish

- Olive oil for drizzling

Instructions:

1. Preheat oven to 375°F (190°C).

2. Layer eggplant, mozzarella, and tomato sauce in a baking dish.

3. Repeat layers, finishing with mozzarella on top.

4. Drizzle with olive oil and bake for 25-30 minutes.

5. Garnish with fresh basil.

Nutrition Information (per serving):

- Calories: 260
- Protein: 12g
- Carbohydrates: 25g
- Fat: 12g
- Fiber: 8g
- Sugar: 10g
- Portion Size: 1 stack

Thai Chicken Lettuce Cups

Ingredients:

- 1 lb ground chicken
- 1 cup water chestnuts, chopped
- 1/4 cup green onions, chopped
- 2 tablespoons low FODMAP soy sauce
- 1 tablespoon lime juice
- Lettuce leaves for cups

Instructions:

1. In a skillet, cook ground chicken until browned.

2. Add water chestnuts, green onions, soy sauce, and lime juice.

3. Cook for an additional 5 minutes.

4. Spoon into lettuce cups.

5. Serve warm.

Nutrition Information (per serving):

- Calories: 220

- Protein: 18g

- Carbohydrates: 15g

- Fat: 10g

- Fiber: 3g

- Sugar: 5g

- Portion Size: 2 cups

Turkey and Avocado Sushi Rolls

Ingredients:

- 4 nori seaweed sheets

- 2 cups sushi rice, cooked

- 1/2 lb turkey breast, sliced
- 1 avocado, sliced
- Pickled ginger and low FODMAP soy sauce for serving

Instructions:

1. Place nori on a bamboo sushi mat.
2. Spread rice evenly over the nori.
3. Arrange turkey and avocado along one edge.
4. Roll tightly, slice, and serve with pickled ginger and soy sauce.

Nutrition Information (per serving):

- Calories: 280
- Protein: 14g
- Carbohydrates: 40g
- Fat: 8g
- Fiber: 6g
- Sugar: 2g
- Portion Size: 8 pieces

Pumpkin and Sage Risotto

Ingredients:

- 1 cup Arborio rice
- 2 cups pumpkin, diced
- 1/2 cup white wine (optional)
- 4 cups low FODMAP vegetable broth
- 1/4 cup fresh sage, chopped
- Parmesan cheese (optional)
- Salt and pepper to taste

Instructions:

1. In a pan, sauté rice until translucent.
2. Add pumpkin and white wine; cook until wine evaporates.
3. Gradually add broth, stirring until absorbed.
4. Stir in sage and cook until rice is creamy.
5. Season with salt and pepper, top with Parmesan if desired.

Nutrition Information (per serving):

- Calories: 300

- Protein: 8g

- Carbohydrates: 50g

- Fat: 6g

- Fiber: 4g

- Sugar: 2g

- Portion Size: 1 cup

Chapter 4: Dinner Recipes

These carefully crafted dishes are not only flavorful but also adhere to the Low FODMAP principles, ensuring a harmonious blend of taste and digestive ease.

Lemon Herb Baked Cod

Ingredients:

- 4 cod fillets
- 2 tablespoons olive oil
- 1 lemon, sliced
- 2 cloves garlic, minced
- 1 teaspoon dried thyme
- Salt and pepper to taste

Instructions:

1. Preheat oven to 375°F (190°C).
2. Place cod fillets on a baking sheet.
3. Drizzle with olive oil and sprinkle with minced garlic, thyme, salt, and pepper.

4. Arrange lemon slices on top of the fillets.

5. Bake for 15-20 minutes or until the cod is flaky.

Nutrition Information (per serving):

- Calories: 250
- Protein: 30g
- Carbohydrates: 2g
- Fat: 12g
- Fiber: 1g
- Sugar: 0g
- Portion Size: 1 fillet

Beef and Vegetable Stir-Fry

Ingredients:

- 1 lb beef sirloin, thinly sliced
- 2 cups broccoli florets
- 1 bell pepper, sliced
- 1 zucchini, sliced
- 3 tablespoons soy sauce (low FODMAP)
- 2 tablespoons sesame oil
- 1 tablespoon ginger, minced

Instructions:

1. Heat sesame oil in a wok or large pan over medium-high heat.
2. Add sliced beef and stir-fry until browned.
3. Add vegetables and ginger, stir-fry until crisp-tender.
4. Pour in soy sauce and toss until everything is well-coated.
5. Serve over cooked rice or quinoa.

Nutrition Information (per serving):

- Calories: 350
- Protein: 25g
- Carbohydrates: 12g
- Fat: 22g
- Fiber: 4g
- Sugar: 3g
- Portion Size: 1.5 cups

Cilantro Lime Chicken with Quinoa

Ingredients:

- 4 boneless, skinless chicken breasts

- 1 cup quinoa
- 1 lime, juiced
- 1/4 cup fresh cilantro, chopped
- 2 tablespoons olive oil
- Salt and pepper to taste

Instructions:

1. Cook quinoa according to package instructions.
2. Season chicken breasts with salt and pepper.
3. In a pan, heat olive oil and cook chicken until golden brown and cooked through.
4. Mix cooked quinoa with lime juice and cilantro.
5. Serve chicken over quinoa.

Nutrition Information (per serving):

- Calories: 420
- Protein: 35g
- Carbohydrates: 30g
- Fat: 15g
- Fiber: 4g
- Sugar: 1g
- Portion Size: 1 chicken breast with quinoa

Eggplant Parmesan (Gluten-Free)

Ingredients:

- 2 large eggplants, sliced
- 1 cup gluten-free breadcrumbs
- 1 cup Parmesan cheese, grated
- 2 cups marinara sauce (low FODMAP)
- 1 cup mozzarella cheese, shredded
- Fresh basil leaves for garnish

Instructions:

1. Preheat oven to 375°F (190°C).
2. Dip eggplant slices in egg, then coat with a mixture of gluten-free breadcrumbs and Parmesan.
3. Place slices on a baking sheet and bake until golden.
4. In a baking dish, layer marinara sauce, baked eggplant, and mozzarella.
5. Repeat layers, ending with a sprinkle of mozzarella.
6. Bake until cheese is bubbly and golden.

Nutrition Information (per serving):

- Calories: 280

- Protein: 12g

- Carbohydrates: 25g

- Fat: 15g

- Fiber: 8g

- Sugar: 10g

- Portion Size: 1 cup

Shrimp and Asparagus Risotto

Ingredients:

- 1 lb shrimp, peeled and deveined

- 1 bunch asparagus, chopped

- 2 cups Arborio rice

- 1/2 cup dry white wine

- 4 cups low FODMAP chicken broth

- 1 cup Parmesan cheese, grated

- 2 tablespoons olive oil

Instructions:

1. In a pan, sauté shrimp until pink, then set aside.

2. In the same pan, add olive oil and sauté asparagus.

3. Add Arborio rice and cook until lightly toasted.

4. Pour in white wine and stir until absorbed.

5. Gradually add chicken broth, stirring until rice is creamy.

6. Stir in cooked shrimp and Parmesan.

Nutrition Information (per serving):

- Calories: 400
- Protein: 20g
- Carbohydrates: 55g
- Fat: 10g
- Fiber: 4g
- Sugar: 2g
- Portion Size: 1 cup

Grilled Pork Chops with Rosemary Potatoes

Ingredients:

- 4 pork chops
- 4 large potatoes, diced
- 2 tablespoons olive oil
- 1 tablespoon fresh rosemary, chopped

- Salt and pepper to taste

Instructions:

1. Preheat grill or oven to medium-high heat.
2. Season pork chops with salt, pepper, and rosemary.
3. Grill or bake pork chops until cooked through.
4. Toss diced potatoes in olive oil, salt, and pepper.
5. Roast potatoes until golden and crispy.

Nutrition Information (per serving):

- Calories: 380
- Protein: 30g
- Carbohydrates: 30g
- Fat: 15g
- Fiber: 4g
- Sugar: 2g
- Portion Size: 1 pork chop with potatoes

Zucchini Noodles with Pesto

Ingredients:

- 4 medium zucchinis, spiralized

- 1 cup cherry tomatoes, halved
- 1/2 cup pine nuts, toasted
- 1/2 cup fresh basil leaves
- 1/2 cup Parmesan cheese, grated
- 2 cloves garlic, minced
- 1/2 cup olive oil
- Salt and pepper to taste

Instructions:

1. In a blender, combine basil, pine nuts, Parmesan, and garlic.
2. With the blender running, slowly add olive oil until smooth.
3. Season with salt and pepper.
4. Toss spiralized zucchini with pesto and cherry tomatoes.

Nutrition Information (per serving):

- Calories: 300
- Protein: 8g
- Carbohydrates: 10g
- Fat: 25g

- Fiber: 4g

- Sugar: 4g

- Portion Size: 2 cups

Moroccan Spiced Chicken Skewers

Ingredients:

- 1 lb chicken breast, cut into chunks

- 2 teaspoons ground cumin

- 1 teaspoon ground coriander

- 1 teaspoon paprika

- 1/2 teaspoon ground cinnamon

- 2 tablespoons olive oil

- Salt and pepper to taste

Instructions:

1. In a bowl, mix cumin, coriander, paprika, cinnamon, olive oil, salt, and pepper.

2. Marinate chicken chunks in the spice mixture for at least 30 minutes.

3. Thread marinated chicken onto skewers.

4. Grill or bake until chicken is cooked through.

Nutrition Information (per serving):

- Calories: 280
- Protein: 30g
- Carbohydrates: 2g
- Fat: 16g
- Fiber: 1g
- Sugar: 0g
- Portion Size: 3 skewers

Teriyaki Salmon with Brown Rice

Ingredients:

- 4 salmon fillets
- 1/2 cup low FODMAP teriyaki sauce
- 2 tablespoons soy sauce (low FODMAP)
- 2 tablespoons honey
- 2 cups cooked brown rice
- Green onions for garnish

Instructions:

1. Preheat oven to 400°F (200°C).
2. In a bowl, mix teriyaki sauce, soy sauce, and honey.

3. Marinate salmon in the mixture for 15 minutes.

4. Bake salmon for 15-20 minutes or until flaky.

5. Serve over cooked brown rice, garnish with green onions.

Nutrition Information (per serving):

- Calories: 380
- Protein: 25g
- Carbohydrates: 40g
- Fat: 12g
- Fiber: 3g
- Sugar: 10g
- Portion Size: 1 salmon fillet with rice

Chicken and Broccoli Casserole (Gluten-Free)

Ingredients:

- 1 lb boneless, skinless chicken breast, cooked and shredded
- 3 cups broccoli florets
- 1 cup lactose-free cheddar cheese, shredded

- 1 cup lactose-free milk
- 2 tablespoons gluten-free flour
- 2 tablespoons butter
- Salt and pepper to taste

Instructions:

1. Preheat oven to 375°F (190°C).
2. In a saucepan, melt butter and stir in gluten-free flour to create a roux.
3. Gradually whisk in lactose-free milk until smooth.
4. Season with salt and pepper, then stir in shredded cheese until melted.
5. In a baking dish, combine shredded chicken, broccoli, and cheese sauce.
6. Bake for 20-25 minutes or until bubbly and golden.

Nutrition Information (per serving):

- Calories: 320
- Protein: 25g
- Carbohydrates: 15g
- Fat: 18g
- Fiber: 3g

- Sugar: 5g
- Portion Size: 1 cup

Spinach and Ricotta Stuffed Chicken Breast

Ingredients:
- 4 chicken breasts
- 1 cup spinach, chopped
- 1 cup lactose-free ricotta cheese
- 1/4 cup Parmesan cheese, grated
- 2 cloves garlic, minced
- Salt and pepper to taste

Instructions:
1. Preheat oven to 375°F (190°C).
2. In a bowl, mix spinach, ricotta, Parmesan, garlic, salt, and pepper.
3. Cut a pocket into each chicken breast and stuff with the spinach-ricotta mixture.
4. Season chicken with salt and pepper.

5. Bake for 25-30 minutes or until chicken is cooked through.

Nutrition Information (per serving):

- Calories: 340
- Protein: 35g
- Carbohydrates: 5g
- Fat: 18g
- Fiber: 2g
- Sugar: 2g
- Portion Size: 1 stuffed chicken breast

Vegetable and Tofu Curry

Ingredients:

- 1 block firm tofu, cubed
- 2 cups mixed vegetables (bell peppers, carrots, zucchini)
- 1 can coconut milk
- 2 tablespoons low FODMAP curry powder
- 1 tablespoon ginger, minced
- 2 tablespoons soy sauce (low FODMAP)

- Fresh cilantro for garnish

Instructions:

1. In a pan, sauté tofu until golden brown.

2. Add mixed vegetables, ginger, and curry powder.

3. Pour in coconut milk and soy sauce, simmer until vegetables are tender.

4. Garnish with fresh cilantro.

Nutrition Information (per serving):

- Calories: 320
- Protein: 15g
- Carbohydrates: 20g
- Fat: 22g
- Fiber: 6g
- Sugar: 4g
- Portion Size: 1.5 cups

Lemon Garlic Shrimp Scampi

Ingredients:

- 1 lb shrimp, peeled and deveined

- 8 oz gluten-free linguine

- 4 tablespoons olive oil

- 4 cloves garlic, minced

- 1/2 cup dry white wine

- Zest and juice of 1 lemon

- Fresh parsley for garnish

- Salt and pepper to taste

Instructions:

1. Cook gluten-free linguine according to package instructions.

2. In a pan, heat olive oil and sauté minced garlic until fragrant.

3. Add shrimp and cook until pink.

4. Pour in white wine, lemon zest, and lemon juice.

5. Toss cooked linguine with shrimp mixture.

6. Garnish with fresh parsley.

Nutrition Information (per serving):

- Calories: 380

- Protein: 25g

- Carbohydrates: 40g

- Fat: 12g

- Fiber: 3g

- Sugar: 2g

- Portion Size: 1.5 cups

Stuffed Bell Peppers with Ground Turkey

Ingredients:

- 4 bell peppers, halved and seeds removed

- 1 lb ground turkey

- 1 cup cooked quinoa

- 1 cup tomato sauce (low FODMAP)

- 1 cup lactose-free cheddar cheese, shredded

- 1 teaspoon Italian seasoning

- Salt and pepper to taste

Instructions:

1. Preheat oven to 375°F (190°C).

2. In a skillet, cook ground turkey until browned.

3. Mix cooked turkey with cooked quinoa, tomato sauce, Italian seasoning, salt, and pepper.

4. Stuff bell pepper halves with the turkey mixture.

5. Top with lactose-free cheddar cheese.

6. Bake for 25-30 minutes or until peppers are tender.

Nutrition Information (per serving):

- Calories: 330

- Protein: 25g

- Carbohydrates: 25g

- Fat: 15g

- Fiber: 5g

- Sugar: 5g

- Portion Size: 2 pepper halves

BBQ Pulled Chicken Lettuce Wraps

Ingredients:

- 1 lb boneless, skinless chicken thighs

- 1 cup low FODMAP BBQ sauce

- 1 tablespoon olive oil

- 1 head iceberg lettuce, leaves separated

- 1 cup shredded carrots

- Green onions for garnish

Instructions:

1. In a slow cooker, combine chicken thighs and BBQ sauce.

2. Cook on low for 6-8 hours until chicken is tender.

3. Shred the cooked chicken using two forks.

4. In a pan, sauté shredded chicken in olive oil until heated through.

5. Spoon pulled chicken into lettuce leaves, top with shredded carrots and green onions.

Nutrition Information (per serving):

- Calories: 280
- Protein: 20g
- Carbohydrates: 20g
- Fat: 12g
- Fiber: 4g
- Sugar: 8g
- Portion Size: 2 lettuce wraps

Chapter 5: Snacks and Appetizers

Welcome to Chapter 5 of our culinary journey, where we explore the delightful world of snacks and appetizers that not only tantalize your taste buds but also adhere to the principles of the Low FODMAP diet.

Parmesan Zucchini Chips

Ingredients:

- 2 medium zucchinis, thinly sliced
- 1/2 cup grated Parmesan cheese
- 1 tablespoon olive oil
- 1 teaspoon garlic-infused oil
- Salt and pepper to taste

Instructions:

1. Preheat the oven to 400°F (200°C).
2. In a bowl, toss zucchini slices with olive oil, garlic-infused oil, Parmesan, salt, and pepper.

3. Arrange slices on a baking sheet and bake for 15-20 minutes until golden and crispy.

4. Enjoy a guilt-free crunchy snack!

Nutrition Information:

- Calories: 120

- Protein: 6g

- Carbohydrates: 8g

- Fat: 8g

- Fiber: 2g

- Sugar: 3g

- Portion Size: 1 serving

Deviled Eggs with Chives

Ingredients:

- 6 hard-boiled eggs, halved

- 3 tablespoons mayonnaise

- 1 teaspoon Dijon mustard

- 1 tablespoon fresh chives, chopped

- Salt and pepper to taste

- Paprika for garnish

Instructions:

1. Scoop out yolks and mash with mayo, mustard, chives, salt, and pepper.

2. Fill egg whites with the yolk mixture.

3. Sprinkle with paprika for a finishing touch.

Nutrition Information:

- Calories: 90

- Protein: 6g

- Carbohydrates: 1g

- Fat: 7g

- Fiber: 0g

- Sugar: 0g

- Portion Size: 2 halves

Greek Yogurt and Dill Dip

Ingredients:

- 1 cup Greek yogurt

- 2 tablespoons fresh dill, chopped

- 1 teaspoon lemon juice

- Salt and pepper to taste

Instructions:

1. Combine Greek yogurt, dill, lemon juice, salt, and pepper in a bowl.
2. Mix well and refrigerate for at least 30 minutes.
3. Serve chilled with your favorite low FODMAP veggies.

Nutrition Information:

- Calories: 60
- Protein: 8g
- Carbohydrates: 4g
- Fat: 2g
- Fiber: 0g
- Sugar: 3g
- Portion Size: 2 tablespoons

Buffalo Chicken Wings

Ingredients:

- 1 lb chicken wings
- 2 tablespoons olive oil

- 1/4 cup hot sauce (check for no FODMAP ingredients)
- 1 tablespoon butter
- Salt and pepper to taste
- Celery sticks for serving

Instructions:

1. Preheat oven to 400°F (200°C).
2. Toss wings in olive oil, salt, and pepper, then bake for 45-50 minutes.
3. In a saucepan, melt butter, add hot sauce, and stir.
4. Coat baked wings in the sauce and serve with celery sticks.

Nutrition Information:

- Calories: 200
- Protein: 15g
- Carbohydrates: 0g
- Fat: 15g
- Fiber: 0g
- Sugar: 0g
- Portion Size: 4 wings

Mozzarella and Tomato Skewers

Ingredients:

- 12 cherry tomatoes
- 12 mini mozzarella balls
- Fresh basil leaves
- Balsamic glaze for drizzling

Instructions:

1. Thread tomato, mozzarella, and basil onto skewers.
2. Arrange on a platter and drizzle with balsamic glaze.

Nutrition Information:

- Calories: 90
- Protein: 5g
- Carbohydrates: 2g
- Fat: 7g
- Fiber: 0g
- Sugar: 1g
- Portion Size: 3 skewers

Roasted Chickpeas

Ingredients:

- 1 can (15 oz) chickpeas, drained and rinsed
- 1 tablespoon olive oil
- 1 teaspoon smoked paprika
- 1/2 teaspoon cumin
- Salt to taste

Instructions:

1. Preheat oven to 400°F (200°C).
2. Toss chickpeas with olive oil, paprika, cumin, and salt.
3. Roast for 30-40 minutes until crispy.

Nutrition Information:

- Calories: 120
- Protein: 5g
- Carbohydrates: 15g
- Fat: 5g
- Fiber: 4g
- Sugar: 0g

- Portion Size: 1/2 cup

Hummus with Carrot Sticks

Ingredients:

- 1 can (15 oz) chickpeas, drained
- 1/4 cup tahini
- 2 tablespoons olive oil
- 1 tablespoon lemon juice
- 1 clove garlic (infused oil for low FODMAP)
- Salt to taste
- Carrot sticks for dipping

Instructions:

1. Blend chickpeas, tahini, olive oil, lemon juice, garlic, and salt until smooth.
2. Serve with carrot sticks for a crunchy and satisfying snack.

Nutrition Information:

- Calories: 100
- Protein: 3g

- Carbohydrates: 10g
- Fat: 6g
- Fiber: 3g
- Sugar: 2g
- Portion Size: 1/4 cup

Cheese and Grape Plate

Ingredients:

- Assorted low FODMAP cheeses (cheddar, brie, swiss)
- Red and green grapes
- Gluten-free crackers

Instructions:

1. Arrange cheeses, grapes, and crackers on a plate.
2. Create an appealing display for a simple and elegant snack.

Nutrition Information:

- Calories: 150
- Protein: 8g

- Carbohydrates: 15g
- Fat: 8g
- Fiber: 2g
- Sugar: 10g
- Portion Size: 1 serving

Bacon-Wrapped Jalapeño Poppers

Ingredients:

- 6 jalapeños, halved and seeds removed
- 12 slices of bacon
- 8 oz cream cheese
- Chives for garnish

Instructions:

1. Fill jalapeño halves with cream cheese.
2. Wrap each with a slice of bacon and secure with a toothpick.
3. Bake at 375°F (190°C) for 20-25 minutes until bacon is crispy.

Nutrition Information:

- Calories: 180
- Protein: 6g
- Carbohydrates: 2g
- Fat: 16g
- Fiber: 0g
- Sugar: 1g
- Portion Size: 2 poppers

Guacamole with Bell Pepper Strips

Ingredients:

- 3 ripe avocados, mashed
- 1 tomato, diced
- 1/4 cup red onion, finely chopped
- 1 tablespoon lime juice
- Salt and pepper to taste
- Bell pepper strips for dipping

Instructions:

1. Mix avocados, tomato, red onion, lime juice, salt, and pepper.

2. Serve with colorful bell pepper strips.

Nutrition Information:

- Calories: 160
- Protein: 3g
- Carbohydrates: 10g
- Fat: 14g
- Fiber: 7g
- Sugar: 2g
- Portion Size: 1/4 cup

Cucumber and Feta Bites

Ingredients:

- 1 cucumber, sliced
- 4 oz feta cheese, crumbled
- Cherry tomatoes, halved
- Fresh mint leaves for garnish

Instructions:

1. Top cucumber slices with crumbled feta.
2. Garnish with cherry tomato halves and mint leaves.

Nutrition Information:

- Calories: 80
- Protein: 4g
- Carbohydrates: 4g
- Fat: 5g
- Fiber: 1g
- Sugar: 2g
- Portion Size: 4 bites

Mixed Nuts and Seeds

Ingredients:

- 1 cup mixed nuts (almonds, walnuts, pecans)
- 2 tablespoons pumpkin seeds
- 1 tablespoon sunflower seeds
- 1 teaspoon olive oil
- Sea salt to taste

Instructions:

1. Toss nuts and seeds with olive oil and sea salt.
2. Roast in the oven at 325°F (163°C) for 15-20 minutes.

3. Let cool before serving.

Nutrition Information:

- Calories: 200
- Protein: 6g
- Carbohydrates: 6g
- Fat: 18g
- Fiber: 3g
- Sugar: 1g
- Portion Size: 1/4 cup

Olive Tapenade on Gluten-Free Crackers

Ingredients:

- 1 cup mixed olives, pitted
- 2 tablespoons capers
- 1 clove garlic (infused oil for low FODMAP)
- 2 tablespoons fresh parsley, chopped
- Gluten-free crackers for serving

Instructions:

1. Pulse olives, capers, garlic, and parsley in a food processor.

2. Spread tapenade on gluten-free crackers.

Nutrition Information:

- Calories: 120
- Protein: 2g
- Carbohydrates: 4g
- Fat: 10g
- Fiber: 2g
- Sugar: 0g
- Portion Size: 2 tablespoons

Edamame with Sea Salt

Ingredients:

- 2 cups edamame, steamed
- Sea salt to taste

Instructions:

1. Steam edamame according to package instructions.

2. Sprinkle with sea salt and toss before serving.

Nutrition Information:

- Calories: 150
- Protein: 12g
- Carbohydrates: 11g
- Fat: 8g
- Fiber: 8g
- Sugar: 3g
- Portion Size: 1 cup

Smoked Salmon Pinwheels

Ingredients:

- 8 oz smoked salmon
- 4 oz cream cheese
- 1 tablespoon fresh dill, chopped
- Cucumber, thinly sliced

Instructions:

1. Mix cream cheese and dill, then spread on smoked salmon.

2. Place cucumber slices and roll into pinwheels.

Nutrition Information:

- Calories: 180
- Protein: 14g
- Carbohydrates: 2g
- Fat: 12g
- Fiber: 0g
- Sugar: 1g
- Portion Size: 4 pinwheels

Chapter 6: Desserts

Each recipe below promises not only a delightful treat for your taste buds but also a mindful choice for those following the Low FODMAP diet. Let's embark on a journey through a variety of desserts that will satisfy your sweet cravings while adhering to your dietary needs.

Chocolate Avocado Mousse

Ingredients:

- 2 ripe avocados
- 1/3 cup unsweetened cocoa powder
- 1/4 cup maple syrup
- 1 tsp vanilla extract
- Pinch of sea salt

Instructions:

1. In a food processor, blend avocados until smooth.
2. Add cocoa powder, maple syrup, vanilla extract, and a pinch of salt. Blend until creamy.

3. Refrigerate for at least 2 hours before serving.

Nutrition Information (per serving):

- Calories: 150
- Protein: 2g
- Carbohydrates: 15g
- Fat: 10g
- Fiber: 6g
- Sugar: 7g
- Portion Size: 1/2 cup

Almond Flour Banana Bread

Ingredients:

- 2 ripe bananas, mashed
- 3 eggs
- 1/4 cup coconut oil, melted
- 1 tsp vanilla extract
- 2 cups almond flour
- 1 tsp baking soda
- Pinch of salt

Instructions:

1. Preheat the oven to 350°F (175°C). Grease a loaf pan.

2. In a bowl, mix mashed bananas, eggs, melted coconut oil, and vanilla extract.

3. Add almond flour, baking soda, and a pinch of salt. Mix until well combined.

4. Pour the batter into the loaf pan and bake for 45-50 minutes.

Nutrition Information (per slice):

- Calories: 180
- Protein: 6g
- Carbohydrates: 12g
- Fat: 14g
- Fiber: 3g
- Sugar: 5g
- Portion Size: 1 slice

Berry and Coconut Ice Pops

Ingredients:

- 1 cup mixed berries (strawberries, blueberries, raspberries)
- 1 cup coconut water
- 1 tbsp maple syrup

Instructions:

1. Blend berries, coconut water, and maple syrup until smooth.
2. Pour the mixture into ice pop molds.
3. Freeze for at least 4 hours before enjoying.

Nutrition Information (per popsicle):

- Calories: 30
- Protein: 1g
- Carbohydrates: 7g
- Fat: 0g
- Fiber: 2g
- Sugar: 5g
- Portion Size: 1 popsicle

Lemon Sorbet

Ingredients:

- 1 cup freshly squeezed lemon juice
- 1/2 cup maple syrup
- 1 cup water

Instructions:

1. Mix lemon juice, maple syrup, and water in a bowl.
2. Pour the mixture into an ice cream maker and churn according to the manufacturer's instructions.
3. Transfer to a container and freeze for 2-3 hours before serving.

Nutrition Information (per serving):

- Calories: 80
- Protein: 0g
- Carbohydrates: 21g
- Fat: 0g
- Fiber: 0g
- Sugar: 18g
- Portion Size: 1/2 cup

Pumpkin Pie Bites

Ingredients:

- 1 cup canned pumpkin puree
- 1/4 cup maple syrup
- 1 tsp pumpkin spice
- 1/2 cup coconut flour
- 1/4 cup chopped pecans

Instructions:

1. In a bowl, mix pumpkin puree, maple syrup, pumpkin spice, and coconut flour.
2. Form into bite-sized balls and roll in chopped pecans.
3. Refrigerate for at least 1 hour before serving.

Nutrition Information (per bite):

- Calories: 70
- Protein: 1g
- Carbohydrates: 9g
- Fat: 3g
- Fiber: 2g
- Sugar: 5g

- Portion Size: 2 bites

Chocolate-Dipped Strawberries

Ingredients:

- 1 pint fresh strawberries
- 4 oz dark chocolate, melted

Instructions:

1. Wash and dry strawberries.
2. Dip each strawberry into melted dark chocolate.
3. Place on a parchment-lined tray and refrigerate until the chocolate hardens.

Nutrition Information (per strawberry):

- Calories: 25
- Protein: 0g
- Carbohydrates: 5g
- Fat: 1g
- Fiber: 1g
- Sugar: 3g
- Portion Size: 3 strawberries

Vanilla Chia Seed Pudding

Ingredients:

- 1/4 cup chia seeds
- 1 cup almond milk
- 1 tsp vanilla extract
- 1 tbsp maple syrup

Instructions:

1. Mix chia seeds, almond milk, vanilla extract, and maple syrup in a jar.
2. Stir well, cover, and refrigerate overnight.
3. Top with your favorite low FODMAP fruits before serving.

Nutrition Information (per serving):

- Calories: 120
- Protein: 4g
- Carbohydrates: 12g
- Fat: 7g
- Fiber: 7g
- Sugar: 3g

- Portion Size: 1/2 cup

Coconut Macaroons

Ingredients:

- 2 cups shredded coconut
- 1/2 cup coconut flour
- 1/2 cup maple syrup
- 1/4 cup coconut oil, melted
- 1 tsp vanilla extract

Instructions:

1. Preheat the oven to 350°F (175°C). Line a baking sheet with parchment paper.
2. In a bowl, mix shredded coconut, coconut flour, maple syrup, melted coconut oil, and vanilla extract.
3. Form the mixture into small mounds on the baking sheet.
4. Bake for 15-18 minutes or until golden brown.

Nutrition Information (per macaroon):

- Calories: 90

- Protein: 1g
- Carbohydrates: 9g
- Fat: 6g
- Fiber: 2g
- Sugar: 6g
- Portion Size: 1 macaroon

Kiwi and Pineapple Fruit Salad

Ingredients:

- 2 kiwis, peeled and diced
- 1 cup fresh pineapple, diced
- 1 tbsp maple syrup
- Fresh mint leaves for garnish

Instructions:

1. In a bowl, combine diced kiwis and pineapple.
2. Drizzle with maple syrup and toss gently.
3. Garnish with fresh mint leaves before serving.

Nutrition Information (per serving):

- Calories: 60

- Protein: 1g
- Carbohydrates: 15g
- Fat: 0g
- Fiber: 2g
- Sugar: 10g
- Portion Size: 1 cup

Raspberry Almond Cake (Gluten-Free)

Ingredients:

- 2 cups almond flour
- 1/2 cup coconut sugar
- 1 tsp baking powder
- 1/2 cup almond milk
- 1/4 cup coconut oil, melted
- 1 tsp almond extract
- 1 cup fresh raspberries

Instructions:

1. Preheat the oven to 350°F (175°C). Grease a cake pan.

2. In a bowl, mix almond flour, coconut sugar, and baking powder.

3. Add almond milk, melted coconut oil, and almond extract. Stir until smooth.

4. Gently fold in fresh raspberries and pour the batter into the cake pan.

5. Bake for 30-35 minutes or until a toothpick comes out clean.

Nutrition Information (per slice):

- Calories: 180
- Protein: 4g
- Carbohydrates: 14g
- Fat: 12g
- Fiber: 3g
- Sugar: 8g
- Portion Size: 1 slice

Mint Chocolate Chip Cookies

Ingredients:

- 2 cups gluten-free all-purpose flour

- 1/2 cup coconut sugar
- 1/2 cup coconut oil, softened
- 2 eggs
- 1 tsp peppermint extract
- 1/2 cup dark chocolate chips

Instructions:

1. Preheat the oven to 350°F (175°C). Line a baking sheet with parchment paper.
2. In a bowl, cream together coconut oil and coconut sugar.
3. Add eggs and peppermint extract, mixing until well combined.
4. Gradually add gluten-free flour, and fold in dark chocolate chips.
5. Drop spoonfuls of dough onto the baking sheet and bake for 10-12 minutes.

Nutrition Information (per cookie):

- Calories: 120
- Protein: 2g
- Carbohydrates: 15g

- Fat: 6g
- Fiber: 1g
- Sugar: 7g
- Portion Size: 1 cookie

Orange Sorbet

Ingredients:

- 1 cup fresh orange juice
- 1/4 cup maple syrup
- 1 cup water
- Zest of one orange

Instructions:

1. In a bowl, mix orange juice, maple syrup, water, and orange zest.
2. Pour the mixture into an ice cream maker and churn according to the manufacturer's instructions.
3. Transfer to a container and freeze for 2-3 hours before serving.

Nutrition Information (per serving):

- Calories: 70
- Protein: 0g
- Carbohydrates: 18g
- Fat: 0g
- Fiber: 0g
- Sugar: 14g
- Portion Size: 1/2 cup

Blueberry Yogurt Popsicles

Ingredients:

- 1 cup lactose-free yogurt
- 1 cup blueberries
- 2 tbsp maple syrup
- 1 tsp vanilla extract

Instructions:

1. In a blender, combine yogurt, blueberries, maple syrup, and vanilla extract.
2. Pour the mixture into popsicle molds and freeze for at least 4 hours.

Nutrition Information (per popsicle):

- Calories: 40
- Protein: 1g
- Carbohydrates: 8g
- Fat: 1g
- Fiber: 1g
- Sugar: 6g
- Portion Size: 1 popsicle

Almond Butter Cups

Ingredients:

- 1/2 cup almond butter
- 1/4 cup coconut oil, melted
- 2 tbsp maple syrup
- 1/4 cup dark chocolate chips

Instructions:

1. In a bowl, mix almond butter, melted coconut oil, and maple syrup.
2. Melt dark chocolate chips in a microwave-safe bowl.

3. Line a mini muffin tin with paper liners. Spoon a small amount of melted chocolate into each cup.

4. Add a spoonful of the almond butter mixture on top of the chocolate and cover with more melted chocolate.

5. Freeze for 2 hours before serving.

Nutrition Information (per cup):

- Calories: 80
- Protein: 2g
- Carbohydrates: 6g
- Fat: 6g
- Fiber: 1g
- Sugar: 4g
- Portion Size: 1 cup

FODMAP-Friendly Apple Crisp

Ingredients:

- 4 cups sliced Granny Smith apples
- 1 tbsp maple syrup
- 1 tsp cinnamon

- 1 cup gluten-free oats
- 1/2 cup almond flour
- 1/4 cup coconut oil, melted
- 2 tbsp chopped pecans

Instructions:

1. Preheat the oven to 350°F (175°C). Grease a baking dish.
2. In a bowl, toss sliced apples with maple syrup and cinnamon. Transfer to the baking dish.
3. In another bowl, mix oats, almond flour, melted coconut oil, and chopped pecans. Sprinkle over the apples.
4. Bake for 35-40 minutes or until the topping is golden brown.

Nutrition Information (per serving):

- Calories: 150
- Protein: 3g
- Carbohydrates: 20g
- Fat: 7g
- Fiber: 4g

- Sugar: 10g
- Portion Size: 1/2 cup

Chapter 7: Smoothies

Embark on a flavorful journey through the vibrant world of smoothies in Chapter 7. These revitalizing concoctions not only satisfy your taste buds but also contribute to your overall well-being.

Berry Blast Smoothie

Ingredients:

- 1 cup mixed berries (strawberries, blueberries, raspberries)
- 1 banana
- 1/2 cup Greek yogurt
- 1/2 cup almond milk
- Ice cubes (optional)

Instructions:

1. Combine mixed berries, banana, Greek yogurt, and almond milk in a blender.
2. Blend until smooth and creamy.

3. Add ice cubes if desired and blend again.

4. Pour into a glass and enjoy!

Nutrition Information:

- Calories: 200

- Protein: 8g

- Carbohydrates: 30g

- Fat: 5g

- Fiber: 6g

- Sugar: 18g

- Portion Size: 1 serving

Green Goddess Smoothie

Ingredients:

- 1 cup spinach

- 1/2 avocado

- 1/2 cucumber

- 1 kiwi

- 1 cup coconut water

- Fresh mint leaves

Instructions:

1. Combine spinach, avocado, cucumber, kiwi, and coconut water in a blender.
2. Add fresh mint leaves for a burst of flavor.
3. Blend until smooth and creamy.
4. Pour into a glass and savor the green goodness!

Nutrition Information:

- Calories: 180
- Protein: 5g
- Carbohydrates: 20g
- Fat: 10g
- Fiber: 8g
- Sugar: 8g
- Portion Size: 1 serving

Tropical Paradise Smoothie

Ingredients:

- 1 cup pineapple chunks
- 1/2 banana
- 1/2 cup mango chunks

- 1/2 cup orange juice
- Coconut flakes (optional)

Instructions:

1. Blend pineapple chunks, banana, mango chunks, and orange juice until smooth.
2. Garnish with coconut flakes for a tropical touch.
3. Blend again briefly.
4. Pour into a glass and transport yourself to a paradise of flavors!

Nutrition Information:

- Calories: 220
- Protein: 3g
- Carbohydrates: 45g
- Fat: 2g
- Fiber: 5g
- Sugar: 35g
- Portion Size: 1 serving

Pineapple Mint Cooler

Ingredients:

- 1 cup fresh pineapple
- 1/2 cup cucumber
- 1 tablespoon fresh mint leaves
- 1/2 lime, juiced
- 1/2 cup coconut water

Instructions:

1. Blend fresh pineapple, cucumber, mint leaves, lime juice, and coconut water until smooth.
2. Adjust mint and lime to taste.
3. Blend again for a refreshing experience.
4. Pour into a glass, and relish the coolness!

Nutrition Information:

- Calories: 150
- Protein: 2g
- Carbohydrates: 35g
- Fat: 1g
- Fiber: 4g

- Sugar: 22g
- Portion Size: 1 serving

Peach and Raspberry Smoothie

Ingredients:

- 1 cup peaches (fresh or frozen)
- 1/2 cup raspberries
- 1/2 cup plain Greek yogurt
- 1/2 cup almond milk
- 1 tablespoon honey (optional)

Instructions:

1. Blend peaches, raspberries, Greek yogurt, almond milk, and honey (if using) until smooth.
2. Taste and adjust sweetness as needed.
3. Blend once more for a velvety texture.
4. Pour into a glass and savor the delightful combination!

Nutrition Information:

- Calories: 220

- Protein: 10g

- Carbohydrates: 30g

- Fat: 6g

- Fiber: 5g

- Sugar: 22g

- Portion Size: 1 serving

Cucumber and Kale Detox Smoothie

Ingredients:

- 1 cucumber

- 1 cup kale leaves, stems removed

- 1/2 green apple

- 1/2 lemon, juiced

- 1 cup coconut water

Instructions:

1. Blend cucumber, kale, green apple, lemon juice, and coconut water until smooth.

2. Adjust lemon juice to taste.

3. Blend once more for a refreshing detox experience.

4. Pour into a glass and rejuvenate!

Nutrition Information:

- Calories: 140
- Protein: 4g
- Carbohydrates: 30g
- Fat: 2g
- Fiber: 7g
- Sugar: 15g
- Portion Size: 1 serving

Chocolate Peanut Butter Banana Smoothie

Ingredients:

- 1 banana
- 2 tablespoons peanut butter
- 1 tablespoon cocoa powder
- 1 cup almond milk
- Ice cubes (optional)

Instructions:

1. Blend banana, peanut butter, cocoa powder, and almond milk until creamy.

2. Add ice cubes if a colder texture is desired.

3. Blend once more for a rich and indulgent treat.

4. Pour into a glass and relish the chocolatey goodness!

Nutrition Information:

- Calories: 280
- Protein: 8g
- Carbohydrates: 30g
- Fat: 16g
- Fiber: 6g
- Sugar: 14g
- Portion Size: 1 serving

Kiwi and Spinach Smoothie

Ingredients:

- 2 kiwis, peeled and sliced
- 1 cup fresh spinach
- 1/2 lime, juiced
- 1/2 cup pineapple juice
- 1/2 cup coconut water

Instructions:

1. Blend kiwis, fresh spinach, lime juice, pineapple juice, and coconut water until smooth.
2. Adjust lime juice to taste.
3. Blend again for a vibrant green delight.
4. Pour into a glass and enjoy the tropical fusion!

Nutrition Information:

- Calories: 160
- Protein: 3g
- Carbohydrates: 35g
- Fat: 1g
- Fiber: 7g
- Sugar: 22g
- Portion Size: 1 serving

Orange Creamsicle Smoothie

Ingredients:

- 1 cup orange segments
- 1/2 cup Greek yogurt
- 1/2 cup almond milk

- 1 tablespoon honey
- Vanilla extract (optional)

Instructions:

1. Blend orange segments, Greek yogurt, almond milk, honey, and vanilla extract until smooth.
2. Adjust sweetness and vanilla to taste.
3. Blend once more for a creamy, dreamy experience.
4. Pour into a glass and reminisce with this nostalgic treat!

Nutrition Information:

- Calories: 180
- Protein: 6g
- Carbohydrates: 25g
- Fat: 4g
- Fiber: 3g
- Sugar: 20g
- Portion Size: 1 serving

Blueberry Almond Butter Smoothie

Ingredients:

- 1 cup blueberries
- 2 tablespoons almond butter
- 1/2 banana
- 1 cup almond milk
- Ice cubes (optional)

Instructions:

1. Blend blueberries, almond butter, banana, and almond milk until smooth.
2. Add ice cubes if a colder consistency is desired.
3. Blend once more for a luscious and nutty experience.
4. Pour into a glass and revel in the blueberry bliss!

Nutrition Information:

- Calories: 250
- Protein: 7g
- Carbohydrates: 30g
- Fat: 12g
- Fiber: 8g

- Sugar: 16g
- Portion Size: 1 serving

Mango Tango Smoothie

Ingredients:

- 1 cup mango chunks
- 1/2 cup pineapple chunks
- 1/2 banana
- 1/2 cup coconut milk
- Fresh mint leaves (optional)

Instructions:

1. Blend mango chunks, pineapple chunks, banana, and coconut milk until smooth.
2. Add fresh mint leaves for a tropical twist.
3. Blend once more for a dance of flavors.
4. Pour into a glass and experience the tango of mango!

Nutrition Information:

- Calories: 220
- Protein: 4g

- Carbohydrates: 35g

- Fat: 8g

- Fiber: 5g

- Sugar: 25g

- Portion Size: 1 serving

Strawberry Coconut Bliss Smoothie

Ingredients:

- 1 cup strawberries

- 1/2 cup coconut flakes

- 1/2 cup plain Greek yogurt

- 1/2 cup almond milk

- 1 tablespoon honey (optional)

Instructions:

1. Blend strawberries, coconut flakes, Greek yogurt, almond milk, and honey until creamy.

2. Taste and add honey if desired.

3. Blend once more for a blissful fusion.

4. Pour into a glass and relish the strawberry coconut symphony!

Nutrition Information:

- Calories: 230
- Protein: 6g
- Carbohydrates: 30g
- Fat: 10g
- Fiber: 7g
- Sugar: 18g
- Portion Size: 1 serving

Papaya Lime Smoothie

Ingredients:

- 1 cup papaya chunks
- 1/2 lime, juiced
- 1/2 cup pineapple juice
- 1/2 cup coconut water
- Ice cubes (optional)

Instructions:

1. Blend papaya chunks, lime juice, pineapple juice, and coconut water until smooth.
2. Add ice cubes for a chilled sensation.

3. Blend once more for a tropical escape.

4. Pour into a glass and transport yourself to the tropics
    with this zesty delight!

Nutrition Information:

- Calories: 170

- Protein: 2g

- Carbohydrates: 40g

- Fat: 1g

- Fiber: 5g

- Sugar: 30g

- Portion Size: 1 serving

Watermelon Mint Refresher

Ingredients:

- 1 cup watermelon cubes

- 1/2 cucumber

- Fresh mint leaves

- 1/2 lime, juiced

- 1/2 cup coconut water

Instructions:

1. Blend watermelon cubes, cucumber, fresh mint leaves, lime juice, and coconut water until smooth.
2. Adjust mint and lime to taste.
3. Blend again for a hydrating and refreshing experience.
4. Pour into a glass and enjoy the revitalizing refresher!

Nutrition Information:

- Calories: 120
- Protein: 2g
- Carbohydrates: 30g
- Fat: 1g
- Fiber: 3g
- Sugar: 20g
- Portion Size: 1 serving

Coffee and Almond Milk Smoothie

Ingredients:

- 1 cup cold brew coffee
- 1/2 banana

- 1/2 cup almond milk
- 1 tablespoon almond butter
- Ice cubes (optional)

Instructions:

1. Blend cold brew coffee, banana, almond milk, and almond butter until smooth.
2. Add ice cubes for an extra chill.
3. Blend once more for a caffeinated delight.
4. Pour into a glass and enjoy the perfect pick-me-up!

Nutrition Information:

- Calories: 160
- Protein: 5g
- Carbohydrates: 20g
- Fat: 8g
- Fiber: 4g
- Sugar: 10g
- Portion Size: 1 serving

CONCLUSION

As we reach the final chapter of this "Low FODMAP Cookbook," it's not just a conclusion but rather an invitation to a new chapter in your culinary journey. The recipes within these pages are more than just delicious meals; they represent a commitment to your well-being, a celebration of flavor, and an exploration of the possibilities within the Low FODMAP framework.

Embarking on the Low FODMAP diet is not merely a dietary choice; it's a pathway to understanding and honoring the intricate relationship between your body and the foods you consume. Each recipe crafted in these pages is a testament to the idea that eating well doesn't mean sacrificing taste or variety. It's about embracing the abundance of nature's bounty and creating dishes that not only adhere to your dietary needs but also tantalize your taste buds.

From the wholesome breakfasts that greet the dawn to the satisfying dinners that cap off your day, this cookbook is a toolbox for crafting meals that resonate with your body's unique rhythms. The 30-day meal plan provides structure, but more importantly, it offers a roadmap for discovering your own culinary preferences within the Low FODMAP landscape.

The snacks, appetizers, desserts, and smoothies aren't mere indulgences; they are the joyful punctuation marks in your daily nourishment, proving that dietary restrictions need not hinder culinary creativity. With a blend of carefully curated ingredients and a dash of imagination, these recipes redefine what's possible within the boundaries of the Low FODMAP diet.

As you delve into these culinary creations, remember that this is not just a cookbook; it's a companion on your journey to health and happiness. It's a guide to savoring every bite, relishing every flavor, and, most importantly, listening to your body's response to the nourishment you provide.

In closing, may this cookbook be more than a collection of recipes — may it be a source of inspiration, a catalyst for discovering new culinary horizons, and a reminder that, with mindful choices and a touch of creativity, you can transform your dietary restrictions into a canvas for delicious and wholesome living. Here's to a future filled with flavorful adventures and the well-deserved joy that comes from nourishing your body, one Low FODMAP bite at a time. Cheers to your health and culinary delight!

www.ingramcontent.com/pod-product-compliance
Lightning Source LLC
Chambersburg PA
CBHW070846260726
48661CB00004B/1256